Medical Management

Principles and Practice

Akmal El-Mazny

Copyright © 2017 Akmal El-Mazny

All rights reserved.

CreateSpace, Charleston SC, USA

ISBN-13: 978-1977697455
ISBN-10: 1977697453

Contents

	PAGE
Introduction	1
Definitions	2
Management Skills	4
Management Principles	6
Management Process	8
−Planning	9
−Implementation	15
−Evaluation	19
Managerial Communication	21
−Understanding Groups	22
−Group Structure	24
−Teamwork	29
−Team Problems	31
Concept of Organization	38
−Organizational Principles	41
Managementm of Time	43
−Steps of Time Management	47
Management of Meetings	55
−Steps of Conducting Meetings	57
Management of Health Systems	70
−Competencies	72
References	75

INTRODUCTION

Management is an art based on science; defined as getting things effectively done to achieve desired objectives through proper planning, efficient implementation, and evaluation.

Planning is the process of formulating objectives and determining the steps that will be employed in attaining them.

Implementation includes: organizing, staffing, directing and leading, coordination of work and team building, recording and reporting, supervision, and monitoring.

Evaluation is intended to measure the degree to which the objectives of the program have been achieved, to identify pitfalls and constraints, and to help re-planning for correction.

Health systems management describes the leadership and general management of hospitals, hospital networks, or health care systems.

This book provides a fundamental knowledge of management principles and practice, emphasizing health systems management, which will be of immense value for all health care professionals.

DEFINITIONS

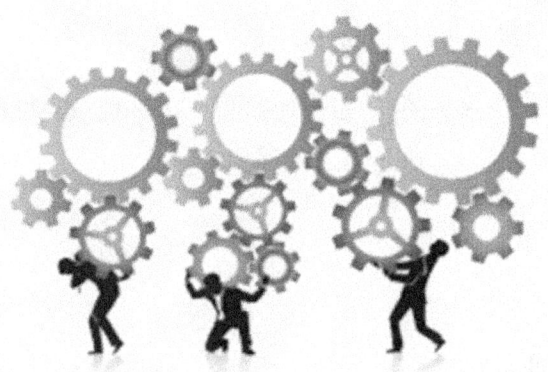

- Management is an art based on science.
- Management is getting things effectively done to achieve desired objectives through proper planning, efficient implementation, and evaluation to identify the needs for re-planning.
- Management is an "interactive process" of administrative and technical functions for the purpose of accomplishing pre-determined objectives through utilization of human and other resources.
- Management is a "decision making process" translating the policies into plans, implementing those plans, and evaluate the plans and the interventions to re-plan to achieve better results.
- Management is a "dynamic process" which should be results-based.

Good Management

– Highlights priorities.

– Makes most of limited resources.

– Adapts services to needs and to changing situations (dynamic).

– Improves the standard and quality of services.

– Maintains high staff morale.

Administration

– Administration is the execution of predetermined policies.

– It represents the implementation element of the management cycle.

Effectiveness

– The degree to which a stated objective is being achieved.

Efficiency

– The optimized use of resources.

MANAGEMENT SKILLS

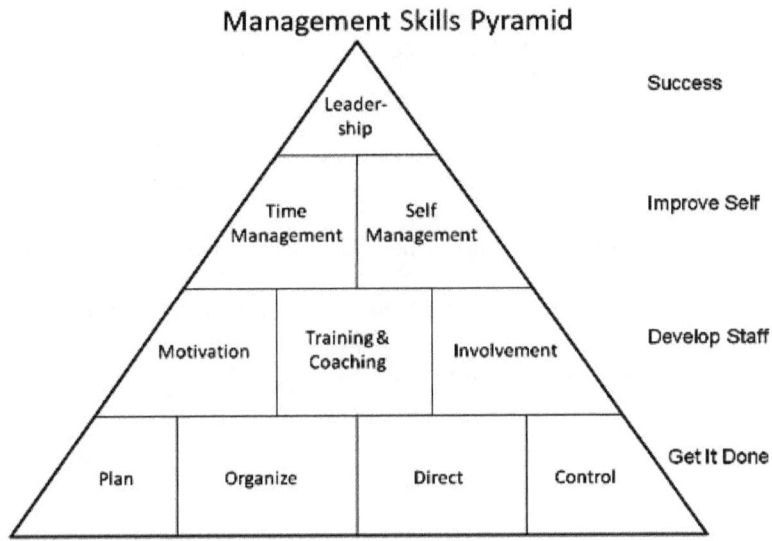

Conceptual Skills

— Ability to understand the complexities of the system, and how the various departments and functions of the organization inter-relate towards convergence of work.

— Ability to understand how the organization relates with the external environment.

Human Skills

– Working with people.

– Ability to communicate effectively with others.

– Ability to motivate and lead people.

Technical Skills

– Ability to use knowledge, methods, techniques and equipment necessary for the the performance of specific tasks acquired from experience, education and training.

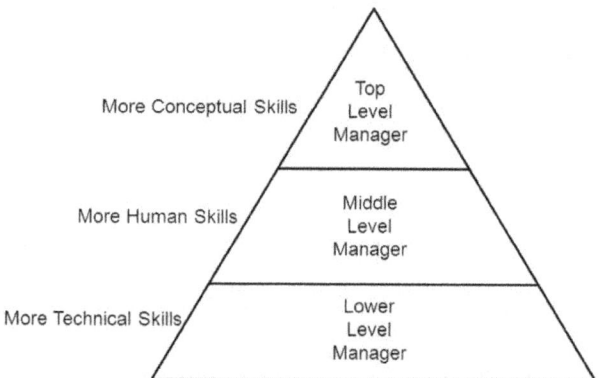

MANAGEMENT PRINCIPLES

Management by Objectives

- Management is getting things done.

- Commitment to achievement.

- Objectives have to be set.

- Means to fulfill these objectives are defined.

- Effectiveness is measured.

Learning from Experience

- If the objectives have not been completely fulfilled, managers ask why?

- What are constraints?

- How to address them?

Division of Labor and Convergence of Work

- Management is getting things done through people.

- To accomplish any activity that needs more than one person, we need two principles:

Division of Labor

− Every body knows his role.

− Division should be done according to the skills of the individuals.

− There must be efficient use of human resources.

Convergence of Work

− Teamwork.

Substitution of Resources

− Management is efficient use of resources.

− Optimizing the use of available resources.

− Maximizing the benefit gained.

− Concept of economy.

Shortest Decision Path

− Decisions have to be made as close as possible, in time and place, to the object of decision and to those affected by it.

− This emphasizes the principles of delegation, decentralization and efficient use of resources.

MANAGEMENT PROCESS

(1) Planning.

(2) Implementation.

(3) Evaluation.

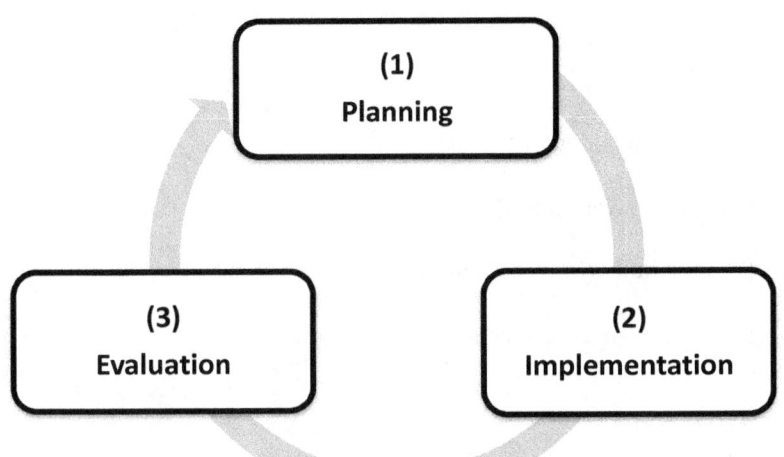

PLANNING

−Planning is the process of formulating objectives and determining the steps that will be employed in attaining them.

−A plan is a statement of goals, objectives and outputs and a description of the courses of action and the resources necessary to achieve them.

Planning Periods

−Long range planning: 3-5 years.

−Yearly plans (work plans).

−A three monthly (implementation plan).

−A Do-it-List (specific executive details).

Levels of Planning

−Top level.

−Middle level.

−First level.

Planning Functions

−Situation analysis.

−Problem identification and priority setting.

−Objectives setting.

−Selection of alternative strategies.

−Planning for resources.

−Planning for monitoring and evaluation.

−Planning for sustainability.

Questions

−Where are we? (Situation analysis).

−Where do we want to go? (Objectives).

−How are we going there? (Plan of action).

−Are we on the right way? (Monitoring).

−Have we reached the objective effectively and efficiently? (Evaluation).

Situation Analysis

The purpose of situation analysis is:

- Identification of different problems, who is suffering from what, where and why, policies and resources.

- To take informed decisions for planning purposes.

Objectives

Should be SMART:

- Specific

- Measurable

- Appropriate / relevant

- Realistic / attainable

- Time-bound

Questions:

- What is going to be accomplished?

- How will it be done?

- When will it be done?

- How much will it cost?

Selection of Alternative Strategies

Criteria for selection:

- Effectiveness.
- Feasibility: technical, financial, social.
- Acceptability.
- Political and institutional support.

Planning for Resources

- Best use of resources.
- Use of alternative resources.

Types of Resources:

- Human.
- Equipment.
- Materials and supplies.
- Money.
- Space.
- Time.
- Information.

Planning for Monitoring and Evaluation

- Monitoring and evaluation must be considered during the planning stage.
- Indicators and criteria to be used have to be well defined.
- Data needs and means for their collection be integrated in the program design.

Planning for Sustainability

A sustainable program is able to:

- Continue its activities.
- Meet its objectives year after year.
- Make plans for the future.
- Fulfill those plans despite changes in outside or inside environment.
- Raise funds so as not to be threatened by loss of a single funding source.

Strategic Planning

− Is the process of determining what an organization intends to be in the future, and how it will get there?

Steps for Strategic Planning

− Mission statement.

− Organization situation analysis (SWOT):

* Strengths.

* Weaknesses.

* Opportunities.

* Threats.

− Identify the problems.

− Establish goals and objectives.

− Select solutions.

− Put an action plan (consider organization stability).

− Implement and monitor the activities.

− Update your plan.

IMPLEMENTATION

- Organizing.

- Staffing.

- Directing and leading.

- Coordination of work and team building.

- Recording and reporting.

- Supervision.

- Monitoring.

Organizing

- It includes organization of all the resources: human power, space, materials, time, and budget.
- The organizing function should thus state: who is going to do what, when, where and how and what is the cost.

Work Plans

- Work plans are needed for all projects, programs, and organizations at all levels: central, governorate, district, and delivery units.

– The work planning process should begin by answering the following questions:

* What are the major activities?
* What is the sequence of the activities?
* Which details of the activities need to be described in the work plan?
* Are the resources available?

Items of Work Plan

– The activities in details.

– The responsible persons.

– Time for implementing the activities.

– Cost (resources).

– Source of funding.

– Work plans are usually done for a period of one year.

The Gant Chart

– The Gant chart is graphic presentation of the time schedule for project or program activities to facilitate implementation and follow up.

Monitoring

– Monitoring is continuous watching over all the resources and day-to-day follow up of the implementation of the planned activities.

– Monitoring is intended to to ensure adequate program operation (work progress, staff performance, and service achievement).

Purpose of Monitoring

Monitoring of Inputs:

– Work progress according to schedule.

– Staff is available.

– Resource consumption and costs are within planned limits.

– The required information is available.

Monitoring of Process:

– The planned functions are performed in accordance with set norms.

– Work standards are met.

– Meetings are held as needed.

– Communication takes place as necessary.

Monitoring of Outputs:

−Products meet specifications.

−Services are delivered as planned.

−Training is effective.

−Decisions are timely and appropriate.

−Records are reliable and reports are issued.

−Conflicts are resolved.

Methods of Monitoring

−Continuous observation.

−Using checklists.

−Examining records.

−Discussing difficulties with staff.

EVALUATION

– Evaluation is a judgment of value based on measuring or assessing the achievements of program activities.

– Evaluation is intended to measure the degree to which the objectives of the program have been achieved, to identify pitfalls and constraints, and to help re-planning for correction.

Methods of Evaluation

– Describe the program to be evaluated.

– Determine the overall goals and specific objectives of the program.

– Identify the indicators to be used.

– Develop the evaluation design.

– Collect data.

– Analyze and interpret these data.

– Utilize the evaluation results in decision making for corrective actions.

Steps of Evaluation

Evaluation of Inputs

– Policies.

– Plans.

– Resources.

– Investments.

Evaluation of Process

– Implementation of activities.

– Limitations.

– Constraints.

Evaluation of Achievements

– The degree to which the objectives have been fulfilled.

MANAGERIAL COMMUNICATION

Group

– Two or more interacting together to achieve particular goals.

Formal Groups

– Work groups defined by the organization's structure that have designated work assignments and tasks.

– Appropriate behaviors are defined by and directed toward organizational goals.

Informal Groups

– Groups that are independently formed to meet the social needs of their members.

UNDERSTANDING GROUPS

Stages of Group Development

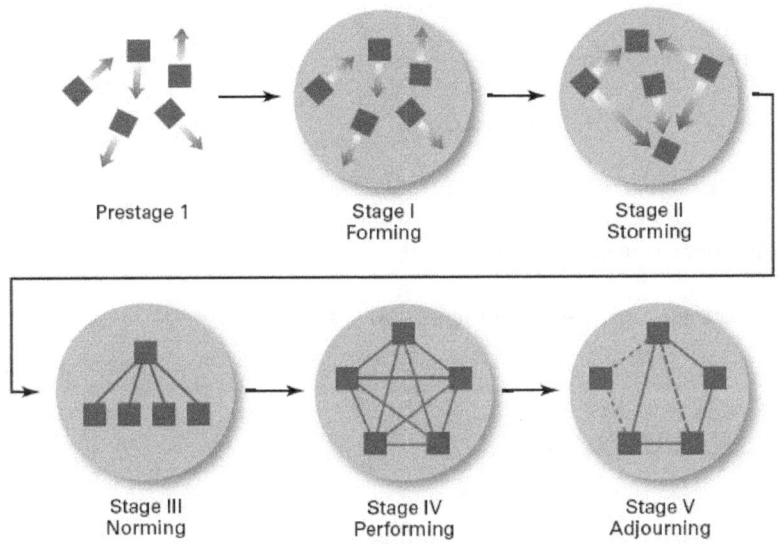

Conditions Affecting Group Behavior

External (Organizational) Conditions

− Overall strategy.

− Authority structures.

− Formal regulations.

− Available organizational resources.

− Organizational culture.

− Employee selection criteria.

− Performance management (appraisal) system.

Internal Group Variables

− Roles.

− Norms.

− Conformity.

− Status system.

− Group size.

− Group cohesiveness.

GROUP STRUCTURE

(1) Roles.

(2) Norms.

(3) Conformity.

(4) Status system.

(5) Group size.

(6) Group cohesiveness.

(1) Roles

− The set of expected behavior patterns attributed to someone who occupies a given position in a social unit that assist the group in task accomplishment or maintaining group member satisfaction.

− Role conflict: experiencing differing role expectations.

− Role ambiguity: uncertainty about role expectations.

(2) Norms

− Acceptable standards or expectations that are shared by the group's members.

Common Types of Norms

−Effort and performance: output levels, absenteeism, promptness, socializing.

−Dress.

−Loyalty.

(3) Conformity

−Individuals conform in order to be accepted by groups.

−Group pressures can have an effect on an individual member's judgment and attitudes.

−Groupthink: the extensive pressure of a strongly cohesive group on individual members to change their opinions to conform to that of the group.

(4) Status System

−Formal or informal.

−Formal status systems are effective when the perceived ranking of an individual and status symbols accorded that individual are congruent.

(5) Group Size

<u>Small Groups</u>

−Complete tasks faster than larger groups.

−Make more effective use of facts.

<u>Large Groups</u>

−Solve problems better than small groups.

−Are good for getting diverse input.

−Are more effective in fact-finding.

<u>Social Loafing</u>

−The tendency for individuals to expend less effort when working collectively than when work individually.

(6) Group Cohesiveness

- The degree to which members are attracted to a group and share the group's goals.
- Highly cohesive groups are more effective and productive than less cohesive groups when their goals aligned with organizational goals.

	Cohesiveness	
Alignment of Group and Organizational Goals	**High**	**Low**
High	Strong Increase in Productivity	Moderate Increase in Productivity
Low	Decrease in Productivity	No Significant Effect on Productivity

Decision Making in Groups

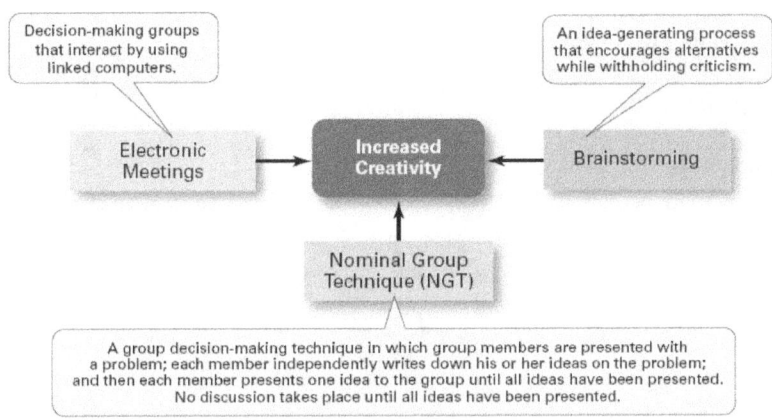

Group Versus Individual Decision Making

Effectiveness	Groups	Individuals
– Accuracy	✓	
– Speed		✓
– Creativity	✓	
– Acceptance	✓	
– Efficiency		✓

TEAMWORK

– Whenever achievement of a common goal needs more than one individual to function together then we need TEAMwork:

* Together.
* Each of us.
* Achieves.
* More.

What Is a Team?

– A group whose members work intensely on a specific common goal using their positive synergy, individual and mutual accountability, and complementary skills.

Advantages of Using Teams

– Teams outperform individuals.

– Teams provide a way to better use employee talents.

– Teams are more flexible and responsive.

– Teams can be quickly assembled, deployed, refocused, and disbanded.

Characteristics of Effective Team

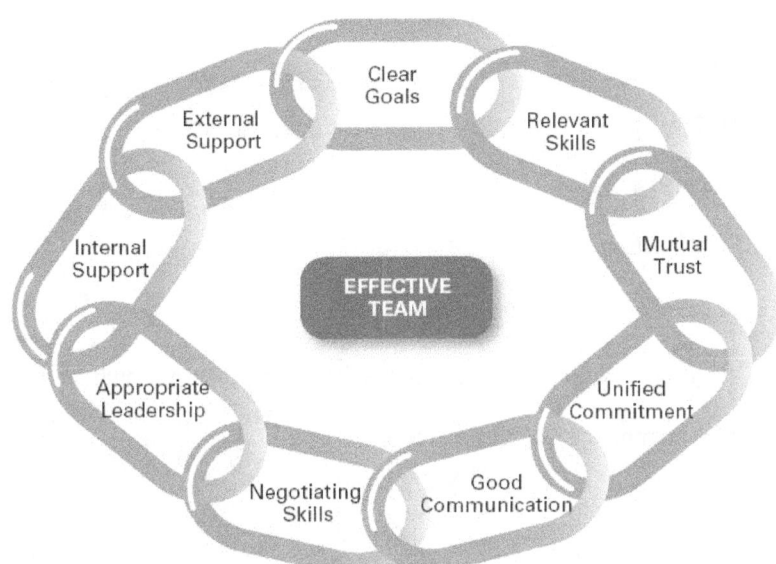

Effective Team Triad

- Treasure.

- Experience.

- Time and effort.

TEAM PROBLEMS

−Problems with:

(1) Goals.

(2) Roles.

(3) Processes.

(4) Relationships.

−These categories represent a hierarchy.

−As we progress down, the problems become more personal and are likely to be more difficult to solve.

(1) Problems with Goals

The potential problems with team goals can be minimized by addressing the following points:

−The goals are clear, specific, measurable, and understood by all the team members.

−The goals are owned and agreed by all the team members.

−The team members have been involved in any development of the initially agreed goals.

(2) Problems with Roles

The problems with roles can be summarized by the extent to which:

- Each team member understands their role and the amount of freedom and authority that they have.
- The different roles of the members fit together without duplicating or missing out tasks.
- If you do not know what game you are playing, how do you know what position to play?

(3) Problems with Processes

Under this large category, there are three broad problem areas:

Decision Making

- Clear responsibility for decision making.
- Levels of authority and rights of veto.
- Who needs to be consulted before decisions are made.
- The extent to which decisions need to be made by consensus.
- How decisions are made in the absence of any individual.
- The ways in which decisions are communicated.

Communication

−What needs to be communicated to whom and by when?

−Balancing communication with information overload.

−Individual tolerances towards being kept fully informed.

Leadership Style

−It is not true that autocrats make poor team leaders or participative managers make good team leaders.

−However, for a team to develop and for a climate of openness and trust to exist, the leader must be prepared to seek and accept feedback on their leadership style, and on the impact it is having on the team.

(4) Problems with Relationships

The problems with relationships are based on the extent to which the individuals in the team:

−Have respect for each other.

−Understand each other.

−Fit together in terms of basic values and attitudes.

Conflict

The perceived incompatible differences in a group resulting in some form of interference with or opposition to its assigned tasks:

- Traditional view: conflict must be avoided.
- Human relations view: conflict is a natural and inevitable outcome in any group.
- Interactionist view: conflict can be a positive force and is absolutely necessary for effective group performance.

Categories of Conflict

- Functional conflicts are constructive.
- Dysfunction conflicts are destructive.

Types of Conflict

- Task conflict: content and goals of the work.
- Relationship conflict: interpersonal relationships.
- Process conflict: how the work gets done.

Handling Conflict

– The role of the manager is not to suppress conflict but to bring it out in a way that allows different opinions to be handled constructively.

Conflict Resolution Techniques

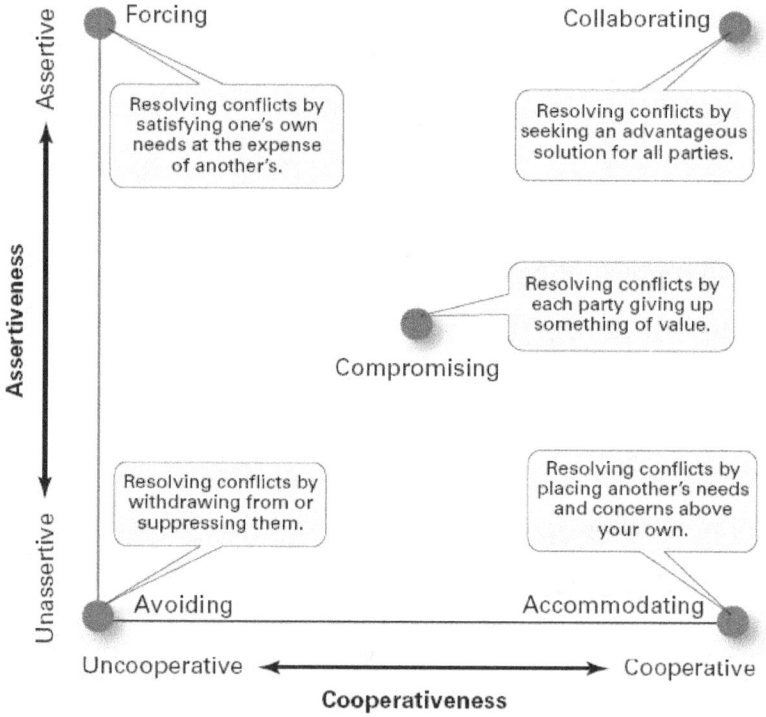

Motivation Process

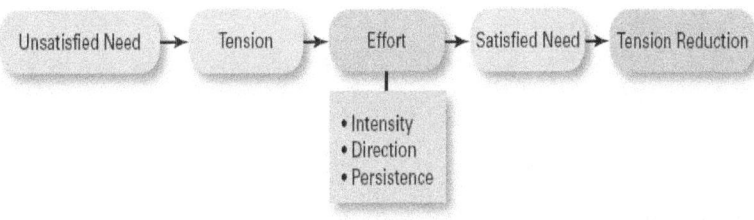

Maslow's Hierarchy of Needs

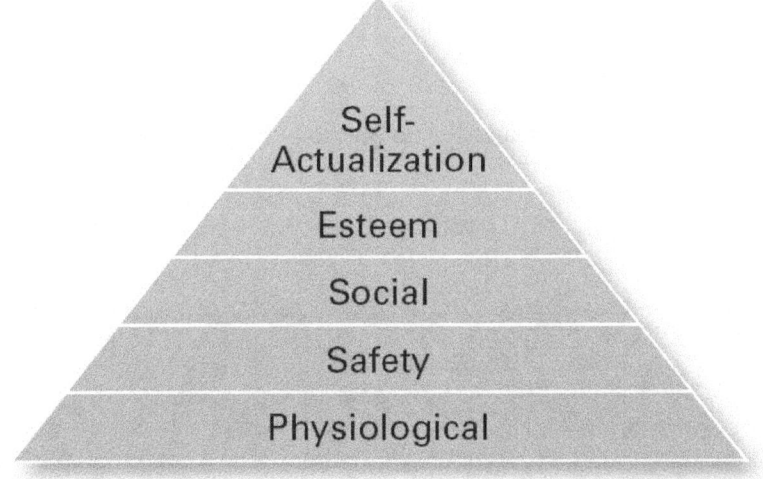

Motivation and Needs

There are three major acquired needs that are major motives in work (Three-need theory):

Need for Achievement (nAch)

— The drive to excel and succeed.

Need for Power (nPow)

— The need to influence the behavior of others.

Need of Affiliation (nAff)

— The desire for interpersonal relationships.

CONCEPT OF ORGANIZATION

- When people come together to combine their talents and efforts, they form organizations.
- Organizations are practices, procedures, and relationships to coordinate human talents and efforts toward common goals.

Working Definition

- Organization is the form of every human association for the attainment of a common purpose.
- The framework of every group moving toward a common objective.
- It refers to the coordination of all these functions as they cooperate for the common purpose.

Reasons for Organizing

- Organizations provide opportunities for accomplishment that are beyond the reach of individuals.
- Effectiveness.
- Efficiency.

Each Organization Should Have

- Clear mission, vision and objectives.

- Work specialization and division of labor.

- Responsibility supported by authority.

- Unity of command.

- Optimum span of control.

Management Functions of an Organization

- Planning: thinking before taking action.

- Organizing: staffing, arranging for material resources, time, and space.

- Coordinating.

- Directing and motivating.

- Controlling.

Organizational Structures

- The hierarchical system.

- The matrix organization.

- Project organization / project teams.

Job Description

– Job title.

– Date.

– Job summary: brief the main responsibilities.

– Duties: detailed description of all activities.

– Relations: accountability and supervision.

– Qualification / job specifications.

– Development: training and career building.

– Job expectations / review / appraisal.

ORGANIZATIONAL PRINCIPLES

− Mission.

− Vision.

− Goals and Objectives.

Mission

− The mission is a statement of purpose.

− What are the main services?

− Who is our customer?

− How do we offer this service?

− Mission is flexible, dynamic, and capable of responding to services as they occur.

Vision

− Describes what the organization hopes to be in the future.

− Spells out the highest ideas and wishes.

− Idealistic aspirations.

− "If you can dream it, you can make it happen".

From Vision to Action

– Vision is transformed into action through an effective strategy.

– Involve people.

– Implement the strategy.

– Measure progress.

Strategy

– A mission is a statement of why an organization exists.

– A vision is a statement of where it's headed.

– A strategy is a statement of how it intends to get there.

Goals and Objectives

– The ultimate desired state towards which objectives and resources are directed.

– The goal is broad, long range, has no timing.

– The goal is related to the organization mission and vision.

MANAGEMENTM OF TIME

Time as a Resource

- Limited resource - we cannot add an hour to the day.
- Cannot be purchased.
- Cannot be replaced (gone is gone).

Habits

- Human beings are creatures of habit.
- We do today what we did yesterday.
- We think today what we thought yesterday.

Definition of Time Management

- The ability of optimal use of time to complete your tasks at a stated / planned time and to live a fruitful, satisfying and enjoyable life.
- A continuous process of analysis, and evaluation of the tasks required in a fixed period of time aiming at maximizing the use of time to achieve stated objectives.

Advantages of Time Management

−Gain time.

−Motivates and initiates.

−Reduces anxiety.

−Self life control.

−Achieve objectives at home, work, family, financial, study, etc.

Need for Good Time Management

−Fulfil objectives and complete tasks at defined times.

−Achieve a balance between work and social life.

−Avoid stress resulting from postponement of work, poor performance, too much of unnecessary work.

Result of Poor Time Management

−Cluttered desks and diaries.

−Cluttered lives.

−Reacting to whatever happens.

−Complain when things go wrong.

Why Do We Loose Control Over Time?

Organizational Factors

−Lack of organizational planning.

−Unclear objectives.

−Lack of clear job descriptions.

−Lack of defined assignments.

−Lack of coordination of work.

−Lack of effective communication.

−Too much paper work.

−Unneeded meetings.

−Lack of delegation.

Social Factors

−Cultural and social norms.

−Social / family problems.

−Social and professional relations.

−Telephone calls / unplanned visits.

Personal Factors

- Lack of motivation.
- Job dissatisfaction, disappointment, etc.
- Psychological / health status.
- Lack of commitment, self discipline.
- Feeling bored, lack of patience.

Environmental Factors

- Poor infrastructure.
- Lack of modern equipments.
- Loss of time to satisfy beraucratic requirements.
- Loss of time in traffic.

STEPS OF TIME MANAGEMENT

(1) Analysis

Analyze How You Spend Your Time

– On long term basis

– On short term basis

Every Second Counts

– Spend every second in an efficient and productive way.

– If you fail to use the day's deposits, the loss is yours.

Negative Views Related to Time

– I do not have time to plan.

– I will be completely devoted to do this task.

– I am the most capable person in doing this.

* I must do every thing by myself.

* Let me do it / OK I will do it.

Discover Your Strengths and Weaknesses

−Interruptions - telephone, personal visitors.

−Un-organized meetings.

−Tasks you should have delegated.

−Acting with incomplete information.

−Dealing with team members.

−Crisis at your work.

−Unclear communication.

−Inadequate technical knowledge.

−Unclear objectives and priorities.

−Lack of planning.

−Stress and fatigue.

−Inability to say "No".

−Desk management and personal disorganization.

−Doing a lot of things at the same time.

−Unclear authorities and responsibilities.

−Lack of work standards and guidelines.

−Perfectionism.

(2) Setting Objectives and Goals

− Where are we? (Situation analysis).

− Where do we want to go? (Objectives).

− How are we going there? (Plan of action).

Personal Objectives and Goals

− Career.

− Community Service.

− Education.

− Exercise.

− Family.

− Finance.

− Friends.

− Spirits.

(3) Maximizing Efficiency in Implementation

Prioritizing

- Prioritizing means determining the relative importance and precedence of events.
- It is absolutely necessary for effective planning.
- Prioritizing keeps us from spending time on things we do not really value.

Circadian Rhythms

- Circadian rhythms are internal biological clocks that regulate many functions and activities; including sleep, alertness, blood pressure, heart rate, temperature, hormone levels, metabolism, and immunity.
- About every 24 hours our bodies cycle through metabolic and chemical changes.
- These circadian rhythms are reset by sunlight each morning.
- Whether you are a "Morning Person" or a "Night Owl" is determined by these cycles.

Owl or Lark?

−Know your best time to work.

−Use that time for priority items.

−Shift natural body clock.

−Change eating schedule.

−Wake with light day.

−Maintain normal routine every day.

Maximize Your Efficiency

−If we learn to listen to our bodies, we can work with these natural rhythms instead of fighting them.

−We can make more efficient use of our time by scheduling certain activities at certain times of the day.

Cognitive Tasks

−Cognitive, or mental, tasks such as reading, calculating, and problem solving are performed most efficiently in the morning.

Short Term Memory

– Short term memory tasks such as last minute reviewing for tests are best performed early in the morning.

Manual Activities

– You are most efficient at tasks involving the use of your hands such as keyboarding and carpentry in the afternoon and early evening.

Physical Workouts

– Because of circadian rhythms, it is best to engage in physical activity in the evening when large muscle coordination is at its peak.
– Studies show the workout to be easier in the evening; exercising about 5 hours before bedtime improves the quality of sleep.

Managing Work Place

– Make your office setting comfortable for your work, and optionally comfortable for others.
– Managing papers: Logic-based papers disposal.
– Managing telephone.

Delegation

– No one is an island.

– You can accomplish a lot more with help.

– People rise to the challenge: You should delegate.

– Grant authority with responsibility.

– Concrete goal, deadline, and consequences.

– Communication Must Be Clear: Get it in writing.

– Trust your people.

Managing Procrastination

<u>We Usually Procrastinate Tasks That</u>

– Produce minimal endorphins.

– Are too lengthy.

– Are too difficult.

– Are too threatening because of the possibility of failure.

– Are too threatening because of the possibility of success.

Steps to Manage Procrastination

−Develop a conditioned response to the tasks you procrastinate.

−Set a goal to complete a task.

−After completing the task, reward yourself with something pleasurable for you; the body releases endorphins - the feel good hormone.

−Over time with repetition, you will come to associate feeling good with completing a task.

−Divide a lengthy task into shorter parts that seem easier to complete.

(4) Monitoring and Evaluation

D.O. I.T. N.O.W.

−D = Divide what you have to do.

−O = Organize your materials, how you will do it.

−I = Ignore interruptions that are distractions.

−T = Take the time to learn how to do things.

−N = Now, not tomorrow.

−O = Opportunity is knocking - Take advantage of opportunities.

−W = Watch out for time.

MANAGEMENT OF MEETINGS

- Meetings are intended to discuss and reach decisions by a group of participants over a specified period of time.
- Meetings need a set of skills.
- They are expensive.
- Meetings take time, human resources involvement, and other resources.
- Meetings can be very useful, or a complete waste of time.
- To be productive meetings must have a Purpose, an Agenda and a Time frame, which is called the PAT approach.

Types of Meetings

There are different types of meetings e.g.:

- Staff meeting: Department meetings, Boards, etc.
- Planning meeting.
- Problem solving meeting.
- Others (conferences and scientific days are considered a sort of a meeting).

People Involved in Meetings Include

- The planner who requests / orders the conduction of the meeting to fulfill certain purpose.
- The facilitator of the meeting who plays the most important role in management of meetings.
- The participants who would be involved in the discussions, decision making and fulfilling the assignments issued from the meetings.

Involved People Should Have

- A clear understanding of the objectives and intended outcomes.
- A clear understanding of the process to be used and confidence in the facilitator who will manage the process.
- A clear understanding of the role of every one attending the meeting.
- Confidence in the utility of the meeting: believe the goal is reachable.
- The opportunity to participate substantively.
- The opportunity to have input to process changes.
- Confidence that follow up will occur and be managed.

STEPS OF CONDUCTING MEETINGS

(1) Selecting participants.

(2) Developing agenda.

(3) Opening the meeting.

(4) Establishing ground rules.

(5) Facilitation of the meeting.

(6) Time management in meetings.

(7) Evaluating the meeting process.

(8) Evaluating the overall meeting.

(9) Closing the meeting.

(10) After the meeting.

(1) Selecting Participants

- To have a successful meeting you should select right people to attend.
- This depends on the purpose of the meeting and the expected actions that will evolve from the meeting.
- Don't depend on a single person opinion; several people may contribute to this selection.
- Some meetings - usually periodic Staff or Board meetings - have a fixed list of participants.
- Guest participants can be invited in a specific meeting according to the purpose of that one in particular.
- If possible, call each person to tell them about the meeting, its overall purpose and why their attendance is important.
- Follow-up your call with a meeting notice, including the purpose of the meeting, where it will be held and when, the list of participants and whom to contact if they have questions.
- Send out a copy of the proposed agenda along with the meeting notice.
- Have someone from the participants "facilitator" designated to record important actions, assignments and due dates during the meeting.

(2) Developing Agenda

- Prepare the Agenda that best use the participant's time and abilities.
- Develop the agenda together with key participants in the meeting.
- Think of what overall outcome you want from the meeting and what activities need to occur to reach that outcome.
- The agenda should be organized so that these activities are conducted during the meeting.
- In the agenda, state the overall outcome that you want from the meeting.
- If the meeting is going to discuss several topics, group them into similar items and make a logical sequence of the topics to be discussed.
- Schedule more difficult topics early in the day, when people have more energy.
- In the agenda state the time of start and end of the meeting, and the time allocated to each item on the agenda.
- Always allow for stretch / bathroom breaks, or coffee breaks at least every two hours.
- Send the agenda of the meeting ahead of time so participants come prepared for the meeting.

(3) Opening the Meeting

- Always start on time; this respects those who showed up on time and reminds late-comers that the scheduling is serious.
- Introduce yourself.
- Welcome attendees and thank them for their time.
- Have the participants introduce themselves.
- This may not be needed if they already know each other.
- If needed, there are three recommended ways depending on:

* How well participants know one another
* How well participants need to know each other, for example:

  Is this the first meeting of a team that needs to develop close relationship?

  Is this a group of people who need to develop enough personal rapport to be able to work collaboratively? Or

  This is a group who will meet just once, with a light task?

* How much time participants will be spending together? Longer meetings generally have more in-depth interactions and require participants to know each other better from the start.
* How much time is available for the introduction?

- Explain the purpose of the meeting; that is the intended outcome, in one sentence if possible.
- Present the objectives of the meeting - Describe what specifically participants are expected to accomplish, in three or four statements.
- Explain the meeting and facilitation approach - What participants can expect to happen in the meeting?
- Review the agenda, giving participants a chance to understand all proposed major topics, change them and accept them.
- Review administrative information - How meals will be handled, where the bathrooms are located, any social activities, any paper work requirements, etc.

(4) Establishing Ground Rules

– Ground rules serve as an informal contract that lays out how things will work and how people will act in the meeting.

– The following are sample of ground rules that may be modified according to the type of meeting and participants:

* Be on time.

* Participate.

* Get focused.

* Maintain momentum.

* Treat all ideas with respect.

* Raise differences openly and constructively.

* Do not interrupt others, ask for the floor if you want to comment.

* No side conversations, always share your ideas with the group.

* Complete the evaluation forms as correctly as you can; this will help improvement in future meetingssss.

* Put your mobile on "Silent".

(5) Facilitation of the Meeting

−A good facilitator follows an "Active Facilitation Approach" to help the group get where they are trying to go and fulfill the purpose of the meeting on time.

Group Discussion

−Discussions can be a creative and productive way to develop a shared understanding of a subject within a group in some depth.

−Discussions are a critical precursor to a group developing a consensus decision where that is a goal.

Advantages of Group Discussions

−Help participants get interested and involved in a subject.

−Enable participants to fill in information gaps and to clear up misunderstandings.

−Enable participants to review and analyze subject matter that has been presented to the group verbally or in writing.

−Identify areas of agreement and disagreement in the group so that differences can be understood and resolved.

Steps of Group Discussions

(1) Prepare for a group discussion:

– Define the objectives of group discussion.

– Develop and write two or three statements / questions to help start and guide the discussions.

(2) Each group will select a group leader and a reporter:

– The group leader will:

* Start and control the discussions to be up to the point keep the time.

* Encourage continued discussions and give the chance for each member to contributes / he will summarize important points.

* Keep the rules of conducting brain storming, if used.

– The reporter will:

* Record discussions and write down important points and conclusions.

* Read to the members the conclusions reached by the group and obtain their approval.

* Present the group report.

(3) Use appropriate group decision-making techniques:

– Brainstorming.

– Nominal Group Technique (NGT).

Brainstorming

(1) Generation phase:

– The question or purpose is clearly noted and written (on a flipchart).

– Responses are invited and recorded (list the ideas).

– Discussion, judgment, and criticism are all suspended during the generation phase.

– A typical generation phase session takes a maximum of 5 to 10 minutes.

(2) Clarification phase:

– The group reviews the list to clarify the meaning of all items or vague terms or statements.

(3) Evaluation phase:

– The brainstorming group reviews the list, eliminates duplications and non-relevant ideas.

– Combine items that seem similar.

– Develop a short list of possible solutions.

Nominal Group Technique (NGT)

– NGT is a group decision-making and problem-solving technique that elicits group members' opinions prior to judgments.

- The technique is particularly effective for setting goals and priorities, and gaining better understanding of complex issues.
- While brainstorming focuses on generating new and creative ideas, the NGT focuses on generating alternatives and selecting among them.
- Conducted within the context of a group meeting, NGT has the following structure:
  * Individuals silently and independently write down their ideas and alternative solutions to a stated problem.
  * All members take turns presenting their ideas, and these ideas are recorded on a flip chart or board.
  * The ideas are discussed only in terms of clarification - evaluative comments are not allowed.
  * A written procedure is followed, which results in a ranking of the alternatives.
- The exact voting procedure is determined in advance, and the winning alternative becomes the selected alternative.
- NGT is a very useful process when there is considerable inhibition, hostility, or a dominant individual.

(6) Time Management in Meetings

—One of the most difficult facilitation tasks is time management - time seems to run out before tasks are completed.

—Therefore, the biggest challenge is keeping momentum to keep the process moving:

* You might ask attendees to help you keep track of the time.

* If the planned time on the agenda is getting out of hand, present it to the group and ask for their input as to a resolution.

—If more is planned for a meeting than time would allow, try:

* Reducing the agenda, for example, by scheduling a second meeting to handle some topics.

* Setting and enforcing short time frames for certain elements.

* Structuring work on several topics concurrently using small groups with clear time limits and specific discussion points to keep them on track.

* Make the meeting a planning session rather than a work session, with tasks to be assigned to follow up sub-teams after the meeting is held.

* Do not deal with time shortages by eliminating or severely restricting discussion time.

(7) Evaluating the Meeting Process

- It is amazing how often people will complain about a meeting being a complete waste of time - but they only say so after the meeting.
- Get their feedback during the meeting when you can improve the meeting process right away.
- Evaluating a meeting only at the end of the meeting is usually too late to do anything about participants' feedback.
- Every couple of hours, conduct 5-10 minutes "satisfaction checks".
- In a round-table approach, quickly have each participant indicate how they think the meeting is going.

(8) Evaluating the Overall Meeting

- Leave 5-10 minutes at the end of the meeting to evaluate the meeting; do not skip this portion of the meeting.
- Evaluation can be anonymous written evaluation or verbal evaluation.
- Have each member rank the meeting from 1-5, with 5 as the highest, and have each member explain their ranking.
- In case of verbal evaluation have chief executive rank the meeting last.

(9) Closing the Meeting

− Always end meetings on time and attempt to end on a positive note.

− At the end of a meeting, review actions and assignments, and set the time for the next meeting and ask each person if they can make it or not (to get their commitment).

− Clarify that meeting minutes or actions will be reported back to members in at most a week (this helps to keep momentum going).

(10) After the Meeting

− Ensure written minutes are prepared and distributed quickly.

− The report should include at a minimum:

* Date:

* Objectives:

* Participants:

* Decisions or outcomes:

* Follow up assignments:

MANAGEMENT OF HEALTH SYSTEMS

Definitions

- Health systems management (or health care systems management) describes the leadership and general management of hospitals, hospital networks, or health care systems.
- The term refers to management at all levels of the health systems.
- Management of a single institution (e.g. a hospital) is also referred to as "medical and health services management", "health care management", or "health administration".

Health Systems Management Ensures That

- Departments within a health facility are running smoothly.
- All departments are working towards a common goal.
- The right people are in the right jobs.
- People know what is expected of them.
- Resources are used efficiently.
- Specific outcomes are attained.

Hospital Administrators

– Hospital administrators are individuals or groups of people who act as the central point of control within hospitals.

– These individuals may be previous or current clinicians, or individuals with other backgrounds.

– There are two types of administrators, generalists and specialists:

* Generalists are individuals who are responsible for managing or helping to manage an entire facility.

* Specialists are individuals who are responsible for the efficient operations of a specific department.

Strengthening Health Systems

The World Health Organization (WHO) proposes that good leadership and management in health need to have a balance between 4 areas:

– Ensuring an adequate number of managers at all levels of health system.

– Ensuring managers have appropriate competences.

– Creating better critical management support systems.

– Creating an enabling working environment.

COMPETENCIES

- The National Center for Healthcare Leadership (NCHL) Model contains three domains - Transformation, Execution, and People - with 26 competencies.

Transformation

- Visioning, energizing, and stimulating a change process that coalesces communities, patients, and professionals around new models of health care and wellness.

Competencies Include

- Achievement orientation
- Analytical thinking
- Community orientation
- Financial skills
- Information seeking
- Innovative thinking
- Strategic orientation

Execution

– Execution is the ability to translate vision and strategy into optimal organizational performance.

Competencies Include

– Accountability

– Change leadership

– Collaboration

– Communication skills

– Impact and influence

– Initiative

– Information technology management

– Organizational awareness

– Performance measurement

– Process management / organizational design

– Project management

People

- Creating an organizational climate that values employees from all backgrounds and provides an energizing environment for them.
- The leader's responsibility to understand his impact on others and to improve his capabilities, as well as the capabilities of others.

Competencies Include

- Human resources management
- Interpersonal understanding
- Professionalism
- Relationship building
- Self confidence
- Self development
- Talent development
- Team leadership

REFERENCES

- Dovlo D. How are we managing? Monitoring and assessing trends in management strengthening for health service delivery in low-income countries. Geneva: World Health Organization (WHO). 2007.
- Egger D, Ollier E. Managing the health Millennium Development Goals-The challenge of management strengthening: Lessons from three countries. Geneva: World Health Organization (WHO). 2006.
- Egger D, Travis P, Dovlo D, Hawken L. Management strengthening in low-income countries. Geneva: World Health Organization (WHO). 2005.
- Frank P. People Manipulation: A Positive Approach. New Delhi: Sterling Publishers. 2009.
- Gomez-Mejia L, Balkin D, Cardy R. Management: People and Performance. Change. New York, USA: McGraw-Hill. 2008.
- Griffin R. CUSTOM Management: Principles and Practices. UK: Cengage Learning. 2014.
- Harris M. Managing Health Services: Concepts and Practice. Marrickville, NSW: Elsevier Australia. 2006.

- Holmes L. The Dominance of Management: A Participatory Critique. Voices in Development Management. Ashgate Publishing. 2012.
- Jones N. The Managerial Culture of Sixteenth-Century England. Jepson Studies in Leadership. Palgrave Macmillan. 2013.
- National Center for Healthcare Leadership (NCHL). Health Leadership Competency Model. National Center for Healthcare Leadership (NCHL). 2005-2010.
- Prasad L, Gulshan S. Management: Principles and Practices. India: Excel Books. 2011.
- Stoner J. Management. Englewood Cliffs, New Jersey: Prentice Hall. 1995.
- Waddington C. Economic and financial management: What do district managers need to know? Geneva: World Health Organization (WHO). 2006.
- World Health Organization (WHO). Building Leadership and Management Capacity in Health. Geneva: World Health Organization (WHO). 2007.

www.ingramcontent.com/pod-product-compliance
Lightning Source LLC
Chambersburg PA
CBHW070318230526
45470CB00002B/937